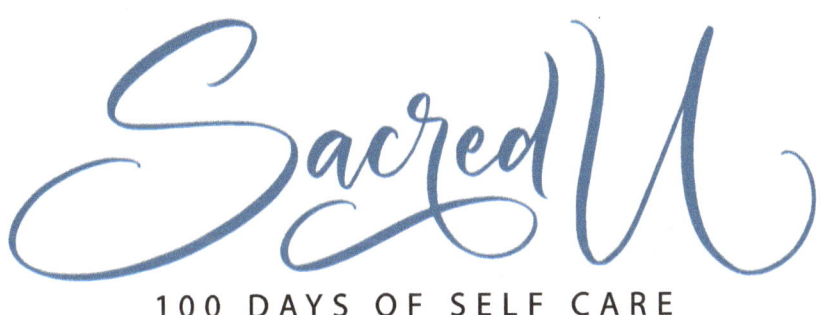

100 DAYS OF SELF CARE

Simple practical activities and inspiring thoughts to support your mind, body and soul.

Anna Russell-Smith

© Anna Russell-Smith 2020

All rights reserved. Except for the quotation of short passages for the purposes of criticism and review, no part of this publication may be reproduced, stored in a retrieval system, or transmitted in any form or by any means, electronic, mechanical, photocopying, recording, or otherwise, without the prior written permission of the Copyright Authority Ltd. or the publisher Innerstar.

Publisher
Innerstar - Mind, Body and Soul
www.innerstar.com.au

Photography
David Russell-Smith

Acknowledgement

With love and thanks to my dad David, for all the beautiful photography work included in this book and for teaching me that everyone has value but not everybody sees it.

ISBN 978-0-6488989-0-0

Dedicated to those souls who've met the black dog.

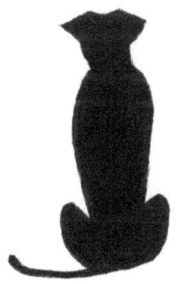

Foreword

Congratulations Anna Smith, an inspiring young lady who has the insight on how to ease the pain of those who are lost within themselves. Her techniques are there to help unlock the pain and anguish suffered by so many. She has achieved so much, my only regret is that 80 years ago there was no Anna Smith for little Mary.

Mary (Maria Tinschert)
Survivor and Author of 'Daughter of the Razor'.

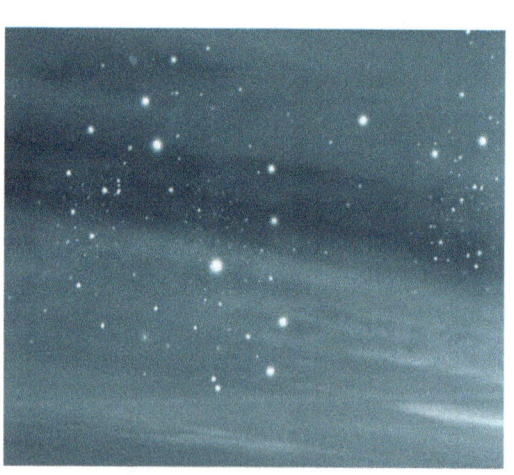

Relax and
watch
the stars...

*Replenish -
walk in nature...*

*Spend time
in a garden...*

Tell someone you love them!

Gratitude –
name three things
to be grateful for...

Read a chapter from a book...

Unplug from technology for the day...

Watch the clouds...
What do you see?

Wear your favourite T-shirt...

Name a strong emotion you have...

Meditate in nature...

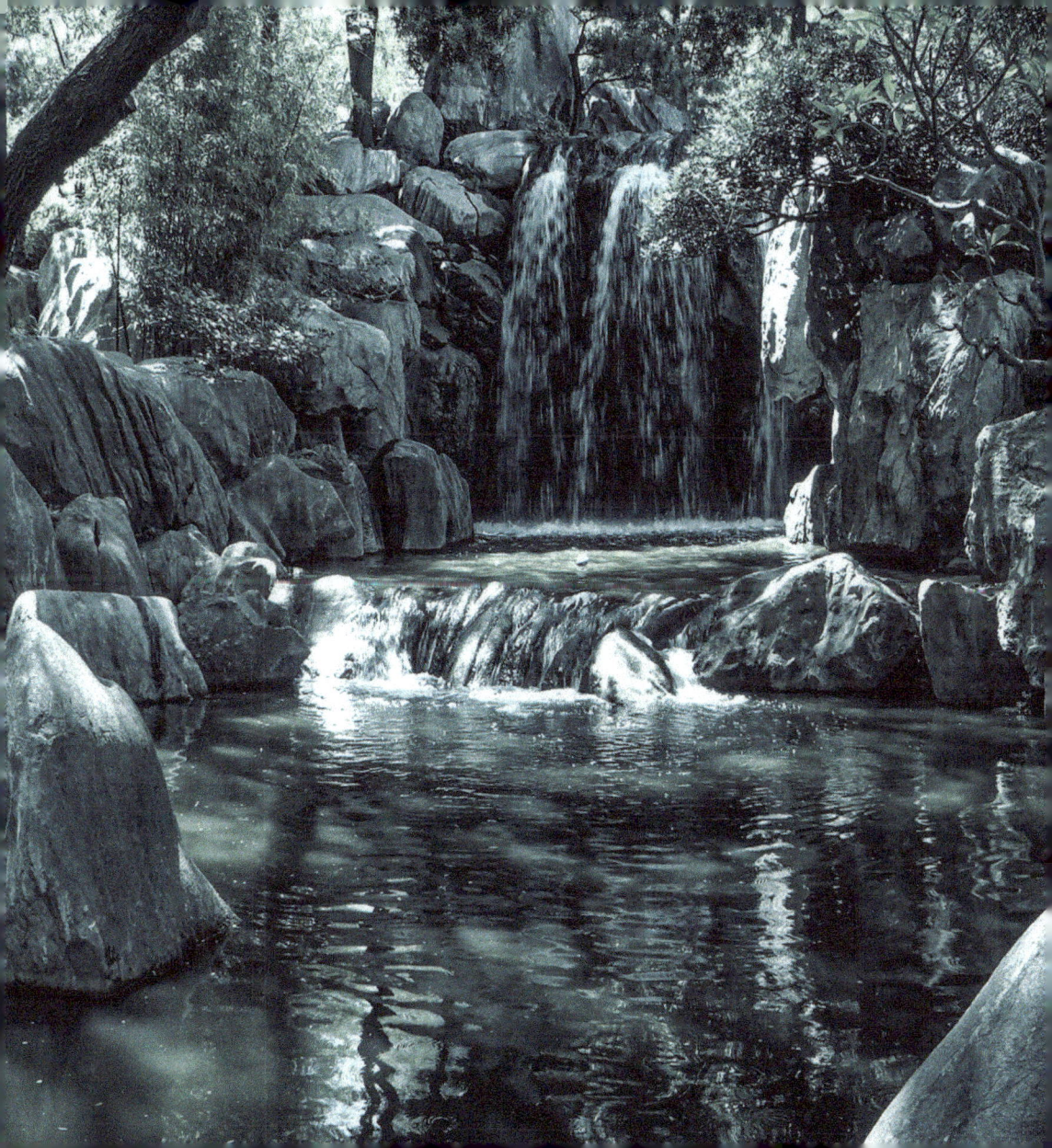

Phone a friend...

Plan a relaxing, evening ritual...

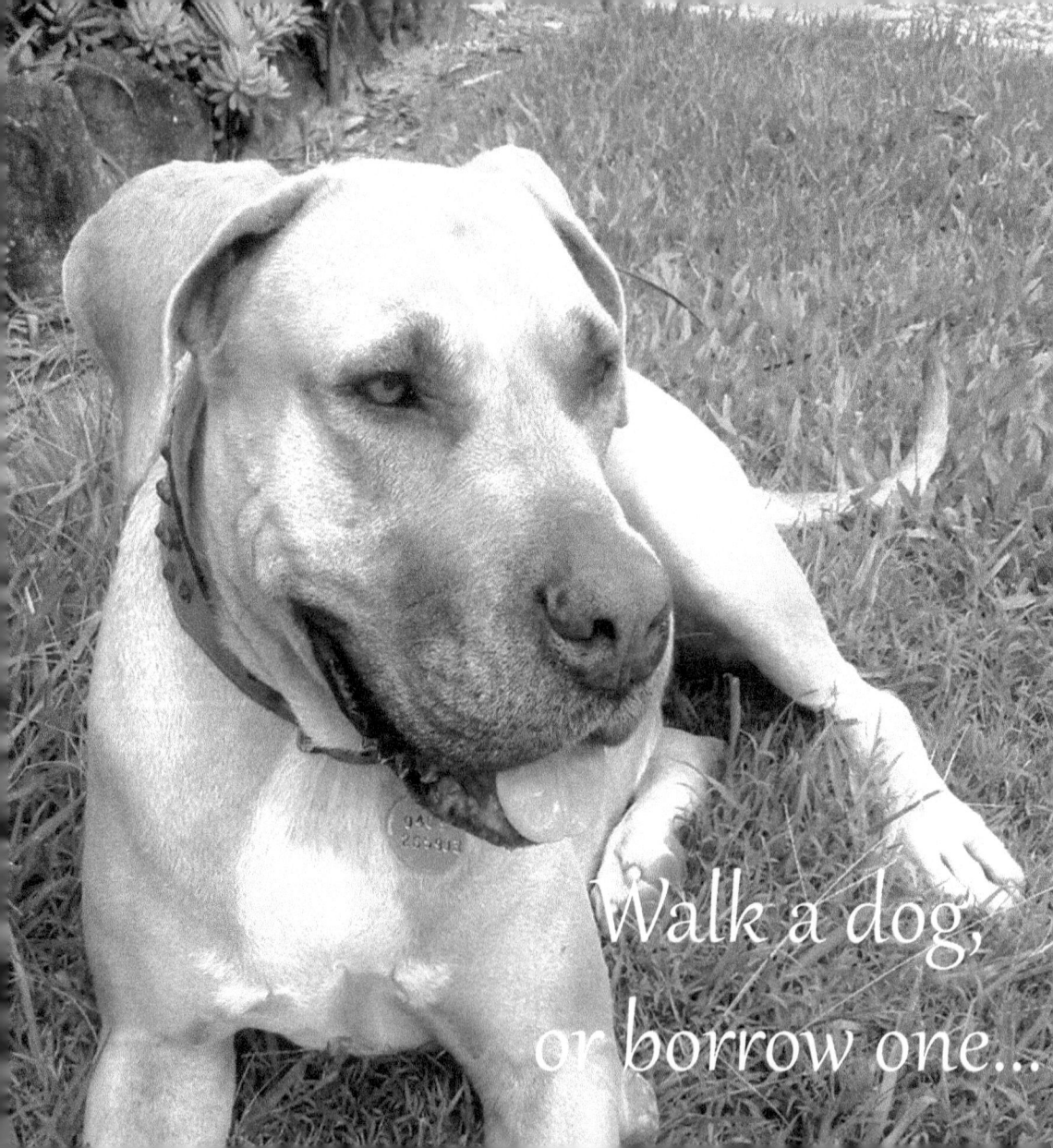

Take a
'you' day...

Pay it forward...

Start a gratitude journal...

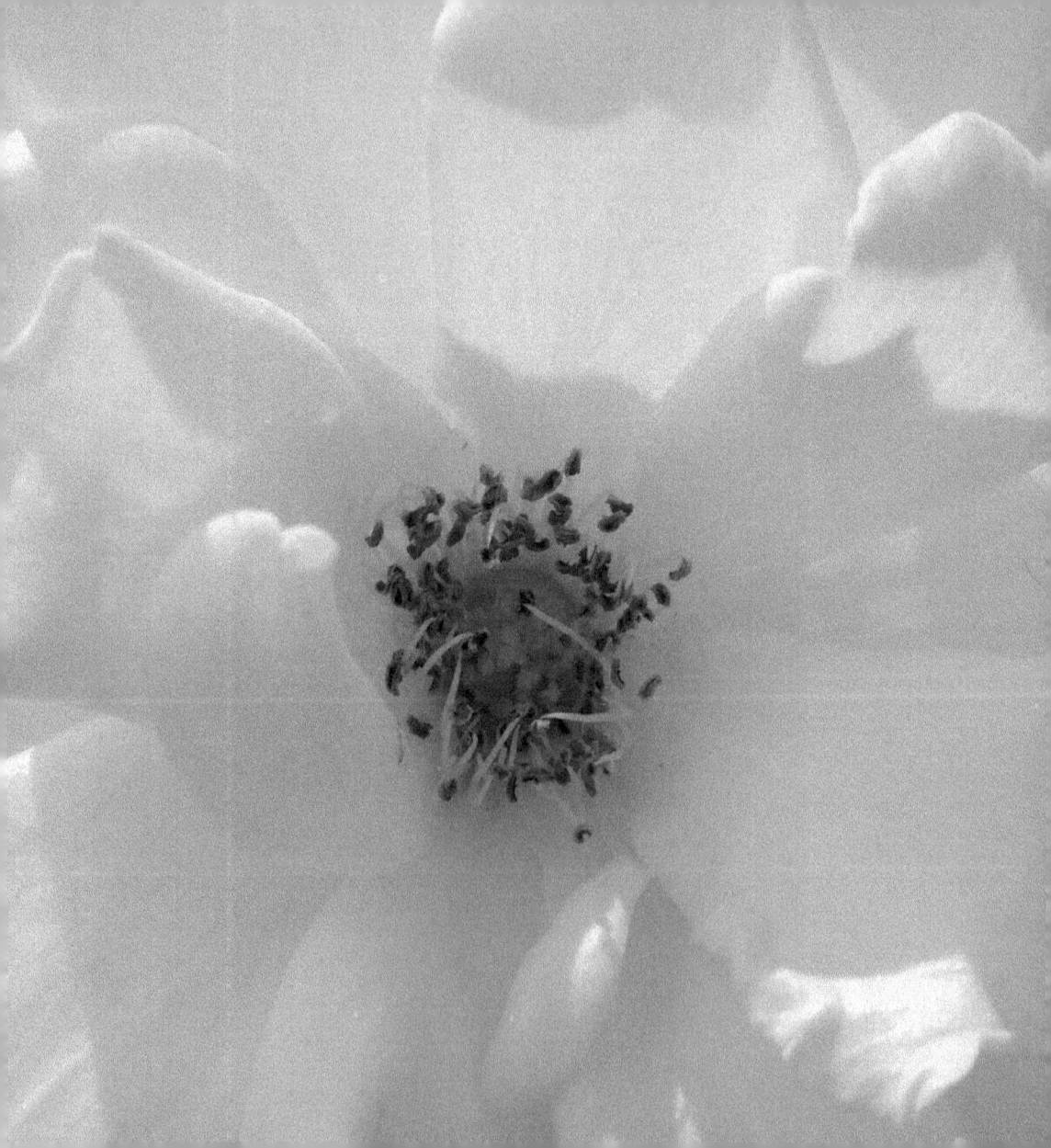

Take a lunch break in nature...

Ask the universe, trust the process...

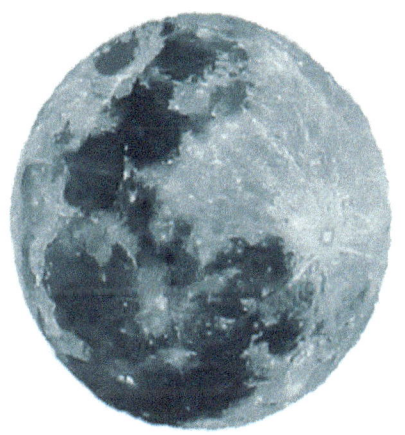

Try a fruit, you've never tasted before...

Soak up some relaxation in a bubble bath...

Pick a flower for someone...

Hydrate, drink plenty of water...

Cook a new healthy recipe...

Honour promises you make to yourself...

Plant a good thought for the day...

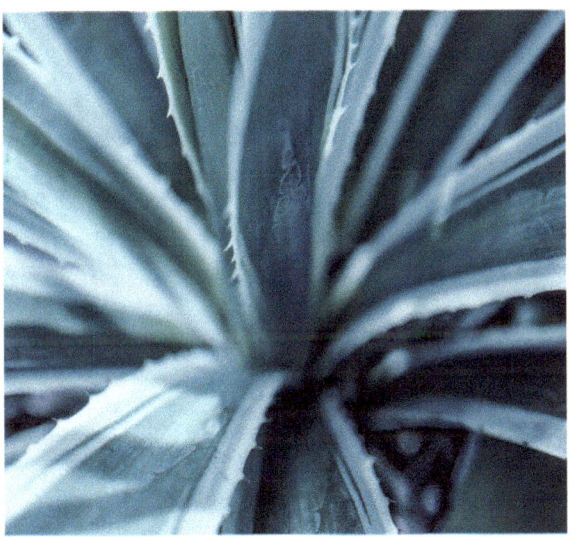

Make a list of all
the wonderful
things about you...

Ground, walk barefoot on the earth...

Download a meditation podcast...

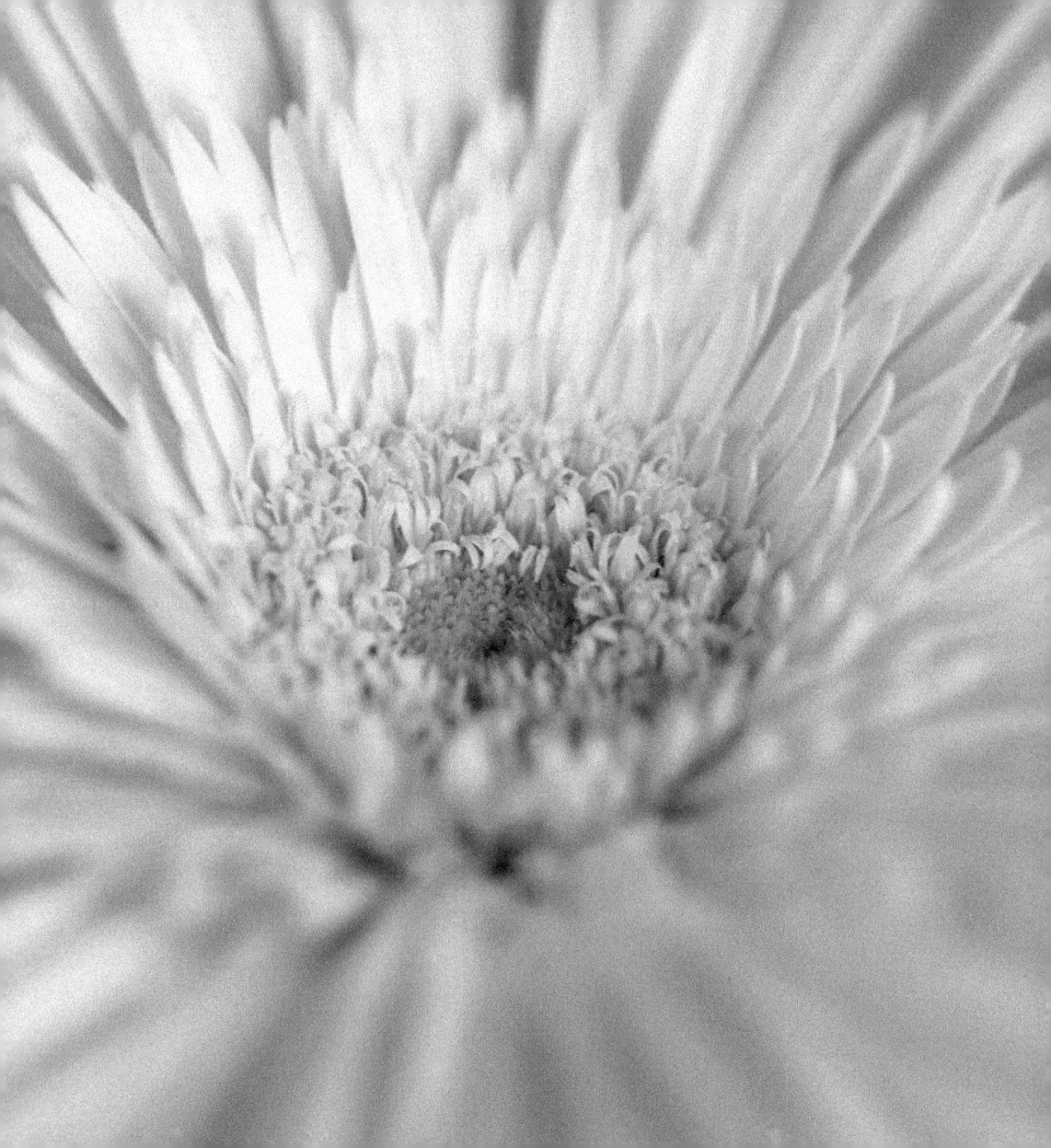

Take a walk on the beach...

Bake something sweet and give away to friends or neighbours...

Write down any worrying thoughts and burn the paper...

Swap a bad habit for something healthy...

Gratitude - name five things you are grateful for...

Plant a seed
from something
you ate...

Connect with a friend...

Like attracts Like...

Make someone

smile...

Visit a library...

Journal your thoughts....

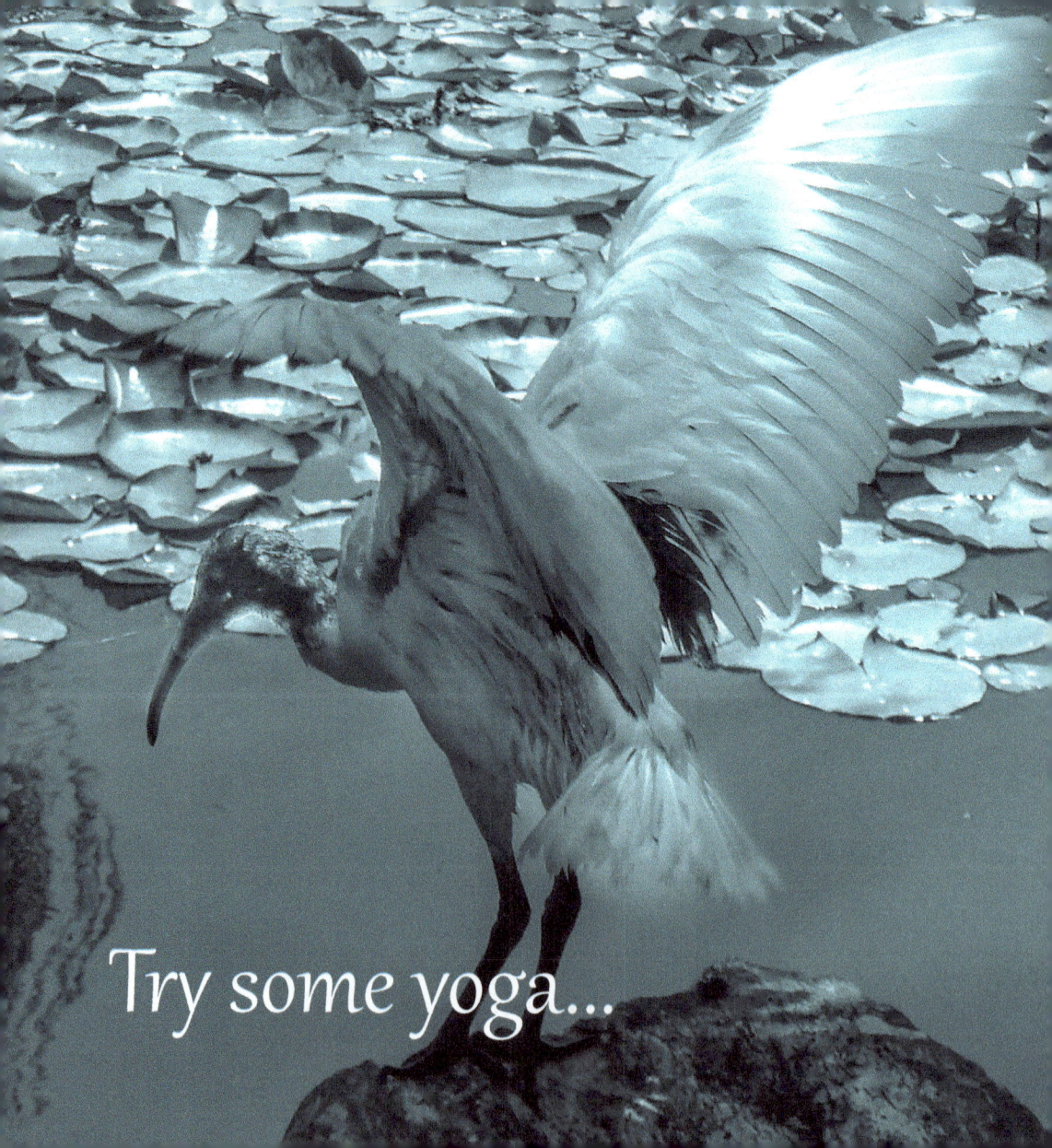

Nurture yourself and others...

Describe the details of a tree...

Make an extra special breakfast...

Share your heart...

Unplug from the digital world for a day...

Meditate in nature...

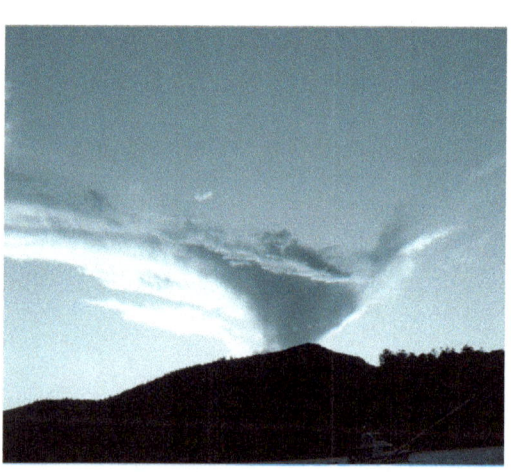

Spend some time in nature...

Work on a small goal for the week...

Gratitude – name six things you are grateful for...

Try a new hairstyle...

Clean out that junk drawer!

Bring the outside in. Pot a plant in a little jar of water...

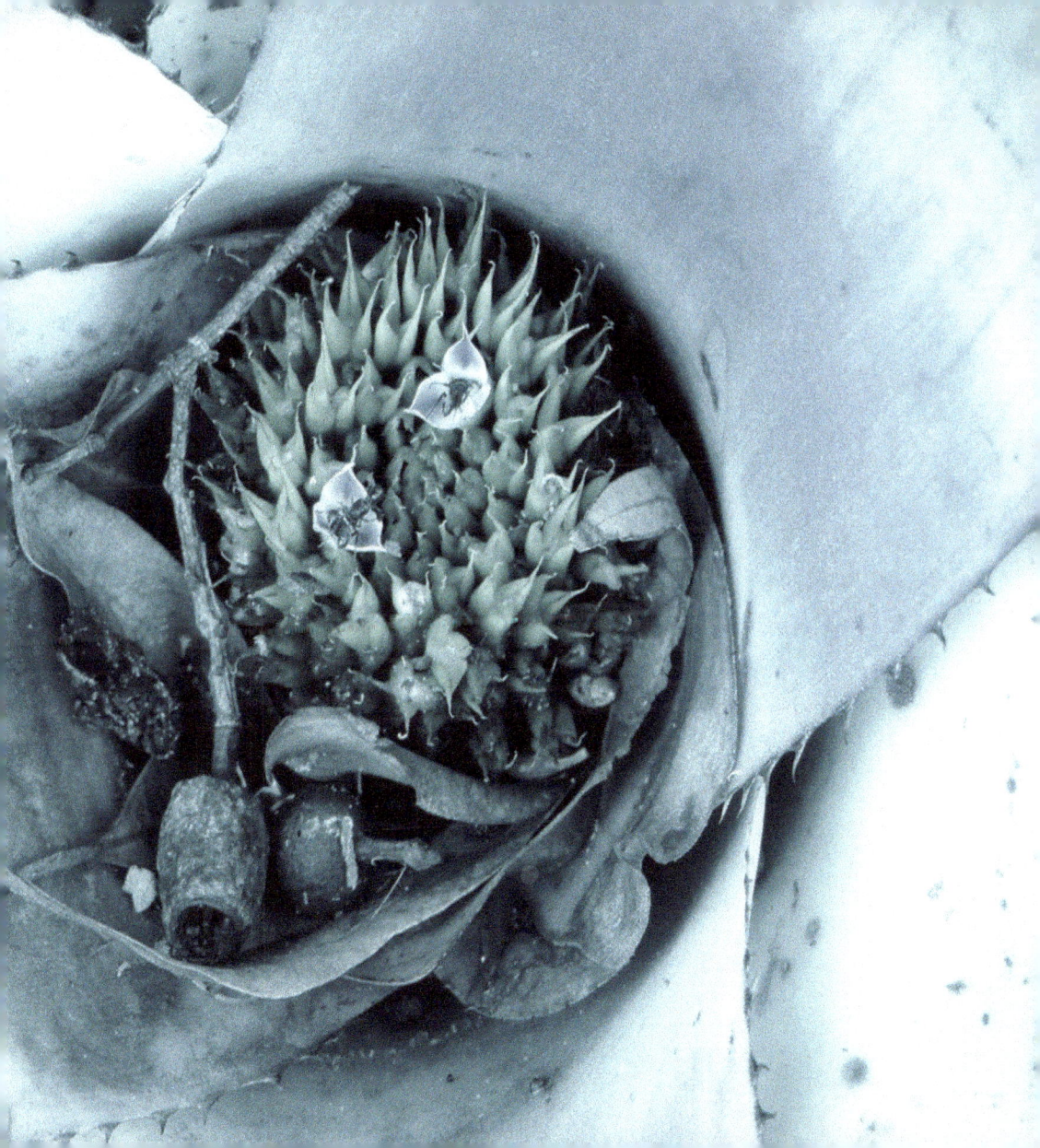

Compliment someone you don't know...

Read a chapter of a book...

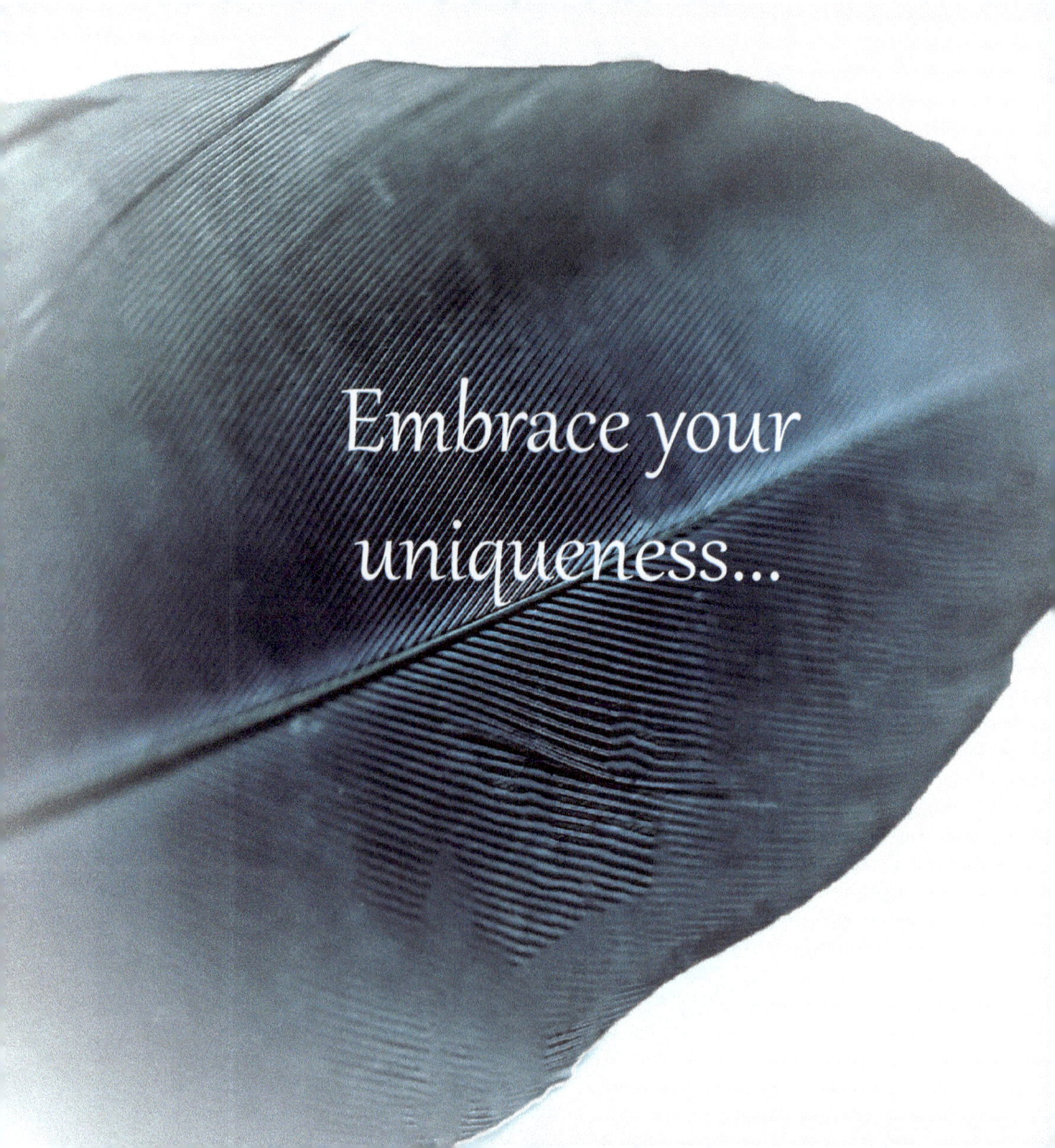

Listen to your favourite music...

Wear your favourite outfit...

Plan a healthy yet delicious recipe...

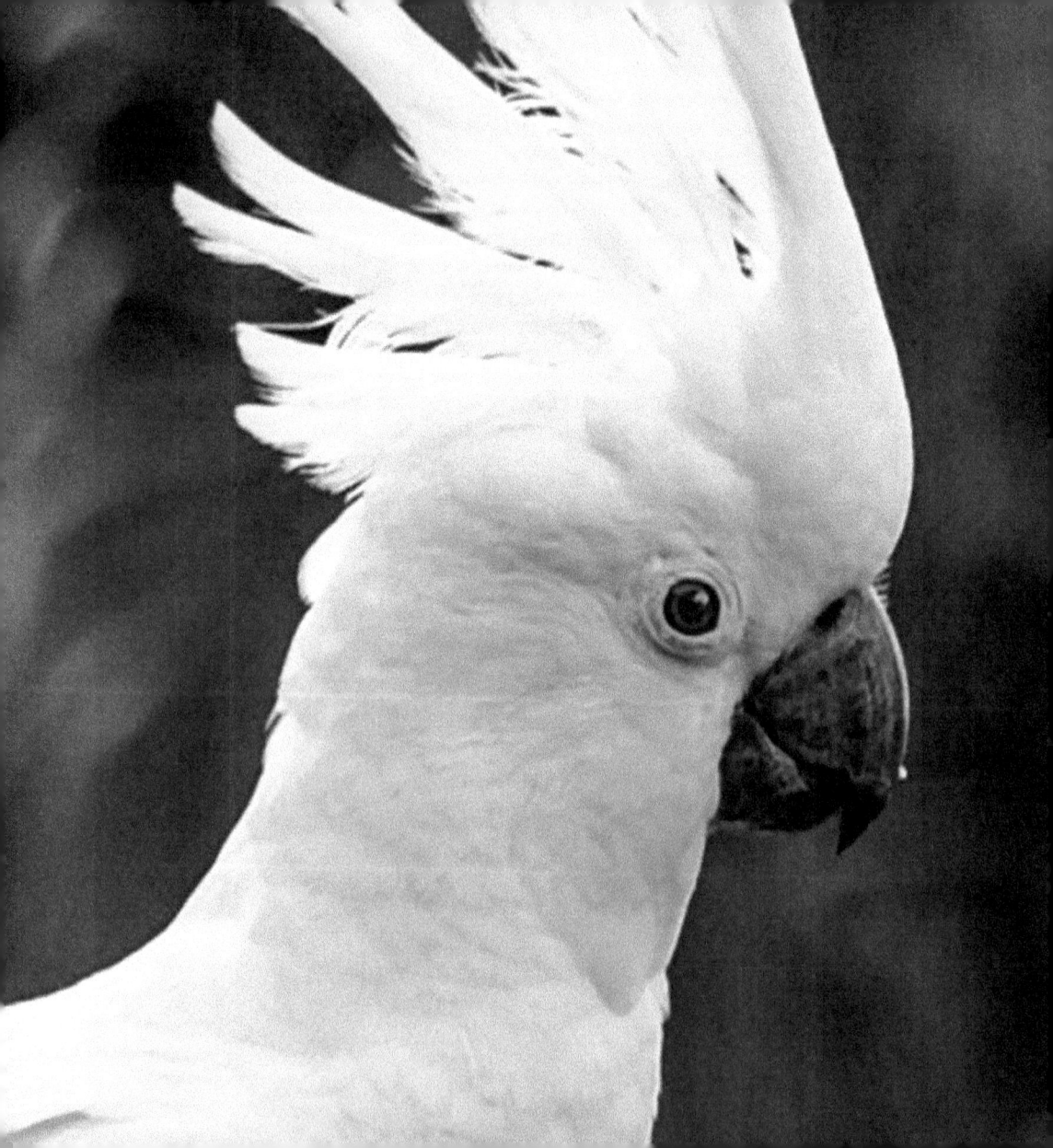

Tell someone close to you what you like about them...

Buy some new underwear...

Rearrange some furniture...

Work on a small
goal for the week...

Spend time in nature...

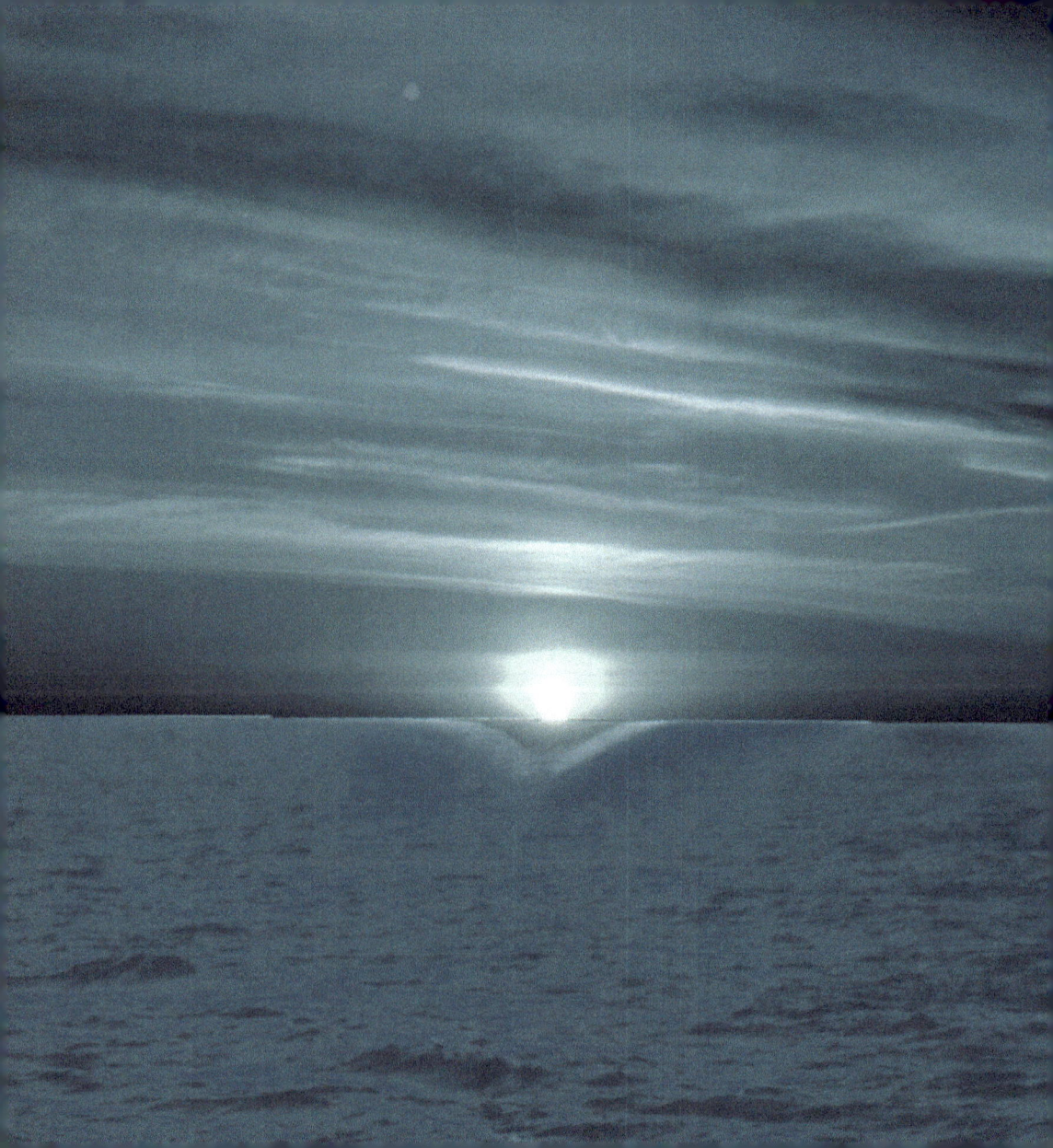

Watch the sunrise or sunset...

Buy a bunch of flowers for yourself, or pick some from your garden...

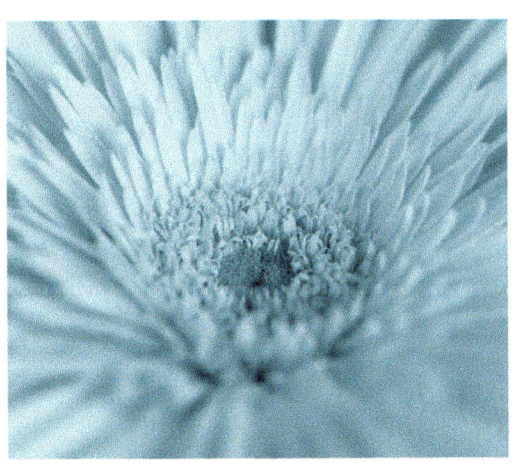

Take a photo of something that captures your eye…

Listen to music
while doing a
household chore...

Gratitude - name three things you are grateful for...

Do something you've put off doing...

Go on a picnic with a friend...

Do a good deed and don't tell anyone about it!

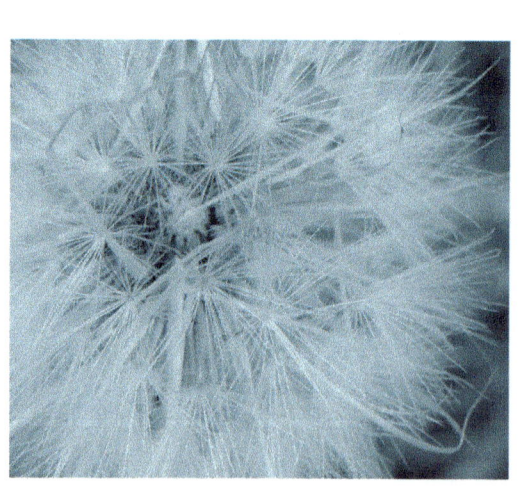

List five things that make you happy...

Make a healthy mocktail and watch the sunset...

Order something at a café you've never tried...

Sing at the top of your lungs...

Spend time in nature...

Throw out five items of clothing you don't wear...

Join a local

meet-up group...

Doing the same thing = same results! What can you change?

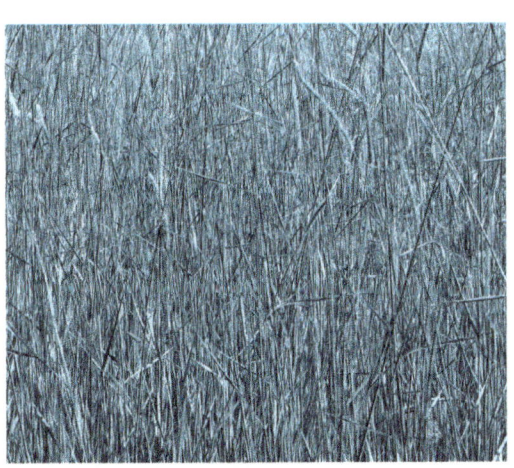

Invest in you...

Read a book...

Celebrate the small wins!

Update your look...

List three short term goals and the steps towards achieving them...

Ask the universe for something for someone else...

Send a surprise care package to someone you care about...

Get creative and paint a picture...

Write a wish list...

Try essential oils...

Walk in nature to nowhere in particular...

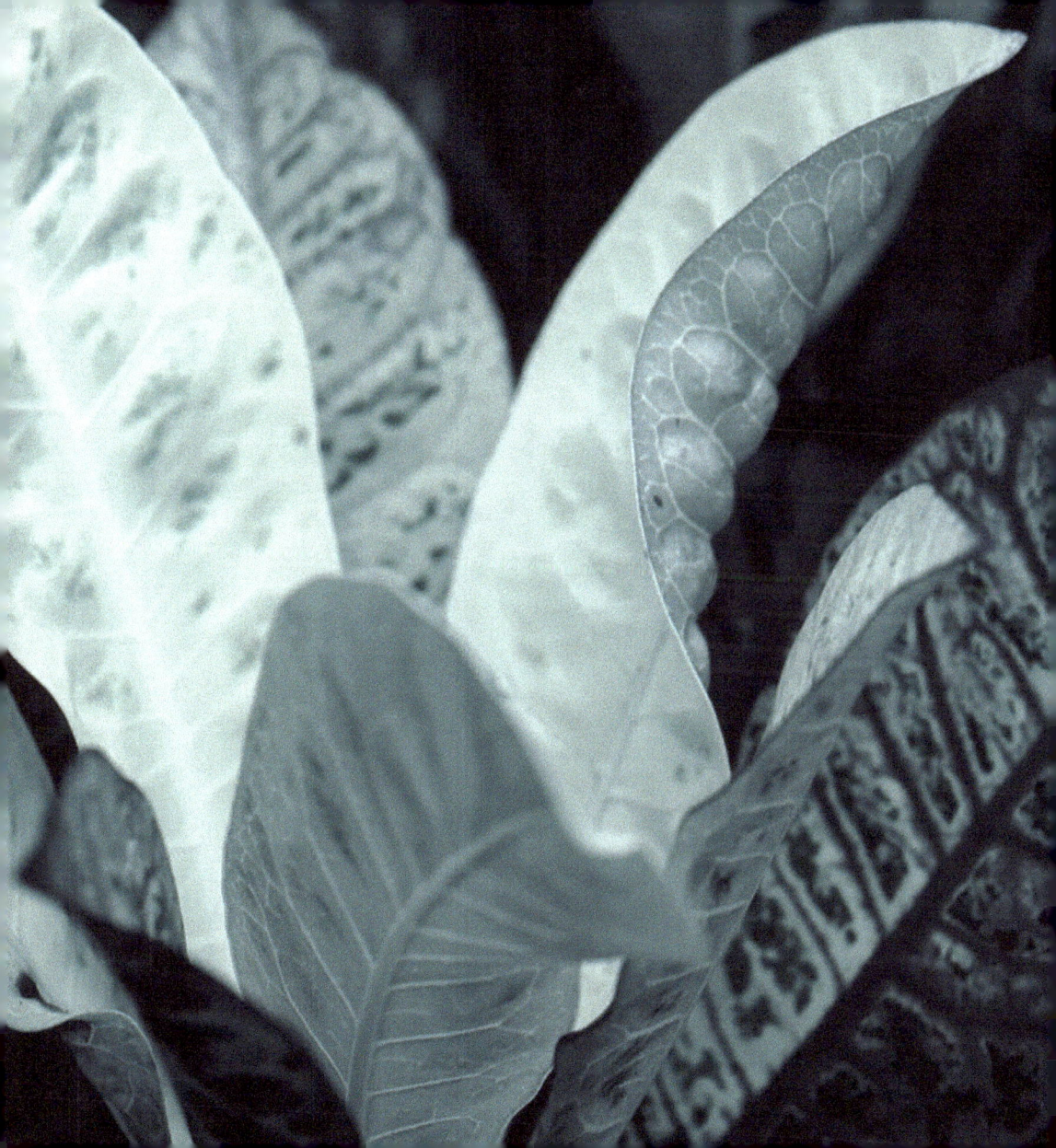

Plan a special treat just for you!

Revisit an old hobby...

Write down who you admire and why...

Listen to a motivational audio book or podcast...

Free hugs to someone just because...

Volunteer at a shelter...

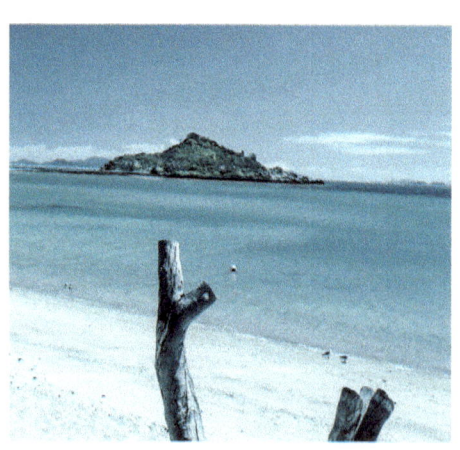

List five long term goals and the steps towards achieving them...

You carry the keys to your dreams...

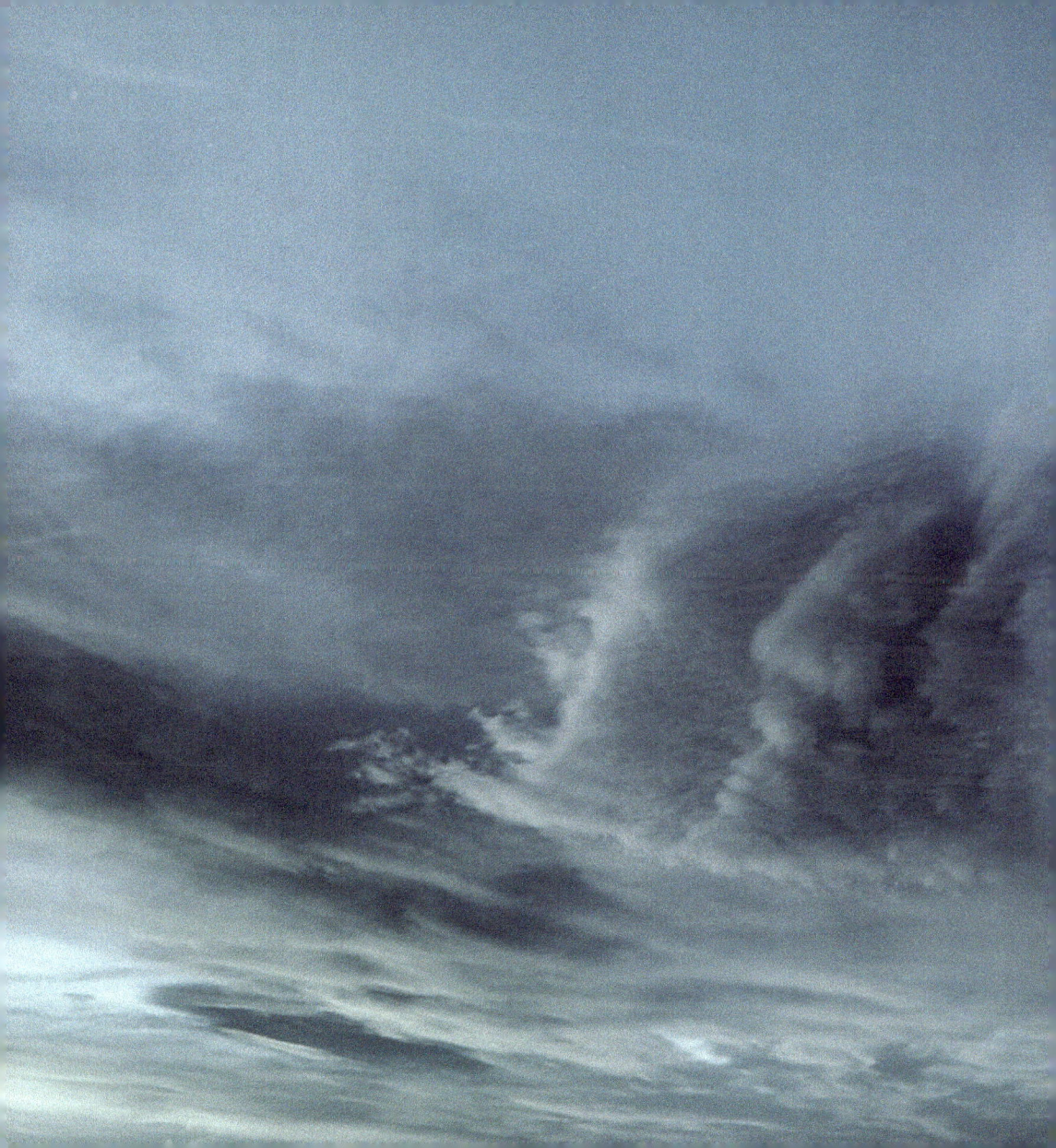

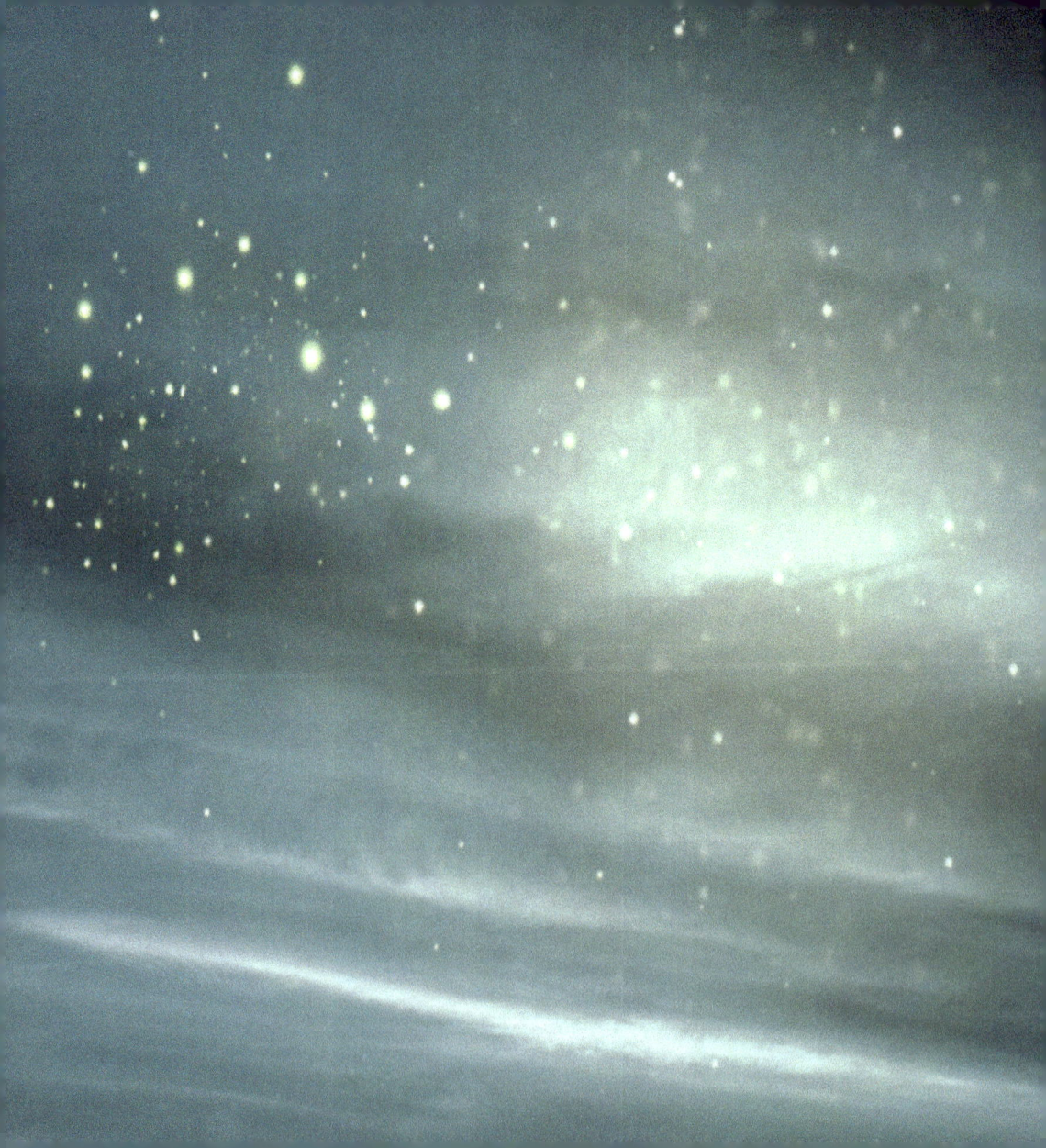

Stargaze and reflect on the last 100 days…

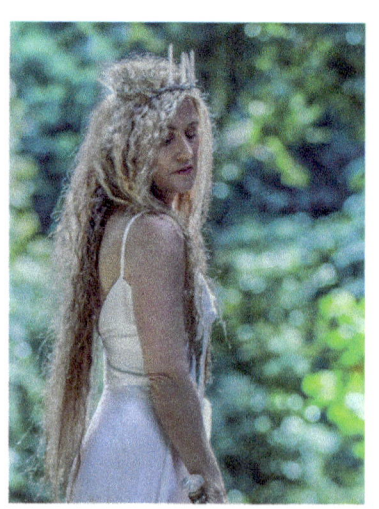

About the Author

Anna Russell-Smith: Clinical Hypnotherapist, Psychotherapist, Counsellor and founder of Innerstar - Mind Body and Soul, based on the Gold Coast, Australia.

With a deep affinity for nature and healing, Anna has been drawn to helping people for as long as she can remember, which led her into the field of counselling for over 15 years.

Anna has supported many people to find their light in times of darkness and uncertainty. Coming from the school of hard knocks herself, she feels this has given her a greater understanding of how to support people to build resilience, self-belief and move forward in life.

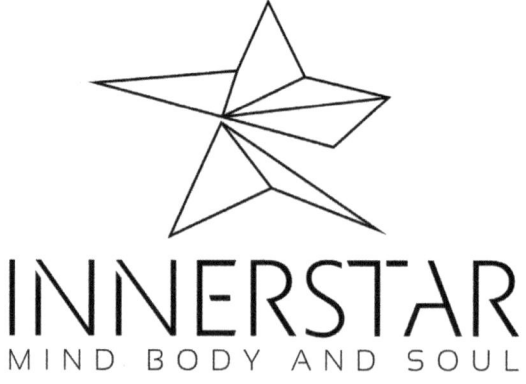

Gold Coast, Australia
www.innerstar.com.au

My gifts to you!

Post a positive review on Amazon or Goodreads, email a screenshot of the review to innerstar6@gmail.com and recieve a complimentary empowerment hypnosis audio download - Sacred U

Mention this book for
10% off online Clinical
Hypnotherapy
or Counselling

Feel you need support?

It's normal to feel sad or worried sometimes, especially when life gets tough. Sometimes, you might need some support to feel better again. If you're struggling with your mental health, support is available. Talk to your GP or health professional, or call Lifeline 24/7 on 13 11 14.

This publication is for information purposes only and is not designed as a treatment for individuals experiencing a mental health condition.

www.ingramcontent.com/pod-product-compliance
Lightning Source LLC
Chambersburg PA
CBHW061133010526
44107CB00068B/2928